2023

LIVER CURE

PROMISING LIVER CURE UNVEILED IN 2023

GARY PAYNE

Copyright © 2023 (GARY PAYNE)

Table Of Content

CHAPTER NINE

123

CHAPTER TEN

139

CHAPTER ELEVEN

145

CONCLUSION 159

INTRODUCTION

In the year 2023, a momentous breakthrough in medical science brought about an extraordinary liver cure, forever altering the landscape of healthcare. This book, "2023 liver cure: promising liver cure unveiled in 2023," delves into the gripping saga of how this revolutionary discovery unfolded. Exploring the intricacies of the liver and the myriad ailments it faces, we uncover the challenges that researchers grappled with for decades. With unwavering determination, they crossed borders, disciplines, and boundaries, fueled by a shared commitment to combat liver diseases. Through the lens of clinical trials, patient experiences, and societal implications, readers bear witness to the profound impact of this life-changing cure. As we traverse the path of hope and resilience, this narrative transcends medical achievements, illuminating the indomitable human spirit in the face of adversity. "2023 Liver cure" invites us to contemplate a future where liver diseases are conquered, and dreams become reality.

CHAPTER ONE

UNDERSTANDING LIVER DISEASES

The liver, a remarkable organ nestled within the human body, plays a vital role in maintaining overall health. It performs a myriad of essential functions, including detoxification, metabolism, and the synthesis of proteins critical for bodily processes. However, like any complex system, the liver is susceptible to a range of diseases that can profoundly impact its functionality.

Liver diseases encompass a diverse array of conditions, each with distinct causes, symptoms, and outcomes. Among the most prevalent are viral infections like hepatitis, autoimmune disorders, fatty liver disease, and cirrhosis. Environmental factors, genetic predispositions, excessive alcohol consumption, and a sedentary lifestyle contribute to the development of these ailments.

Understanding liver diseases necessitates a comprehensive exploration of their pathophysiology, diagnosis, and treatment. Early detection through routine screenings and awareness of potential risk factors are crucial in mitigating the impact of these conditions. Medical professionals, through innovative research and technological advancements, continue to seek effective treatments and potential cures for these life-altering diseases.

Moreover, fostering public awareness about liver health and adopting preventive measures are imperative in curbing the rising incidence of liver diseases. Education on lifestyle modifications, vaccination against viral infections, and responsible alcohol consumption can significantly reduce the burden of liver-related ailments.

In this journey to comprehend liver diseases, we unearth the complexities of this organ's resilience and vulnerabilities. This understanding serves as a foundation for progress in medical research, compassionate patient care, and ultimately, the pursuit of a healthier future. Together, as we deepen our knowledge and awareness, we hold the key to empowering individuals and communities in safeguarding their liver health and well-being.

Anatomy and Function of the Liver

Nestled beneath the rib cage, the liver is the largest internal organ in the human body. Its intricate anatomy and multifaceted functions make it a true powerhouse, playing a vital role in sustaining life. Situated on the right side of the abdomen, the liver consists of four lobes: the right, left, quadrate, and caudate lobes. Within its structure, a complex network of blood vessels, bile ducts, and hepatocytes (liver cells) collaborate to perform an array of essential functions.

Metabolism lies at the core of the liver's responsibilities. It regulates carbohydrate, lipid, and protein metabolism, aiding in nutrient absorption and distribution throughout the body. The liver acts as a storage depot for glycogen, releasing glucose when the body requires an energy boost. Additionally, it synthesizes cholesterol, triglycerides, and essential proteins like albumin and clotting factors.

Detoxification is another critical role performed by the liver. It filters and metabolizes toxins, drugs, and other harmful substances, protecting the body from potential harm. This detoxification process involves two phases, where enzymes convert harmful compounds into water-soluble substances that can be excreted via bile or urine.

The liver's contribution to the digestive process is also indispensable. It produces bile, which is stored in the gallbladder and released into the small intestine to aid in the breakdown and absorption of dietary fats. Bile also aids in the body's elimination of waste.

Moreover, the liver plays a pivotal role in the immune system. Kupffer cells, a type of specialized macrophage within the liver, act as sentinels, identifying and neutralizing pathogens and foreign particles that enter the bloodstream.

Regeneration is one of the most astounding features of the liver. Even when damaged, it has the unique ability to regenerate and restore its functionality, making it a remarkable organ for self-repair.

The interconnected functions of the liver make it a critical hub for maintaining homeostasis and overall health. Its multifaceted nature has earned it the title of the body's metabolic factory. Understanding the anatomy and function of the liver is crucial for appreciating its significance in human physiology and the pivotal role it plays in ensuring our well-being.

Common Liver Disorders

One of the most prevalent liver disorders is non-alcoholic fatty liver disease (NAFLD). NAFLD is a condition characterized by the accumulation of excessive fat in the liver, not caused by alcohol consumption. It encompasses a spectrum of liver diseases, ranging from simple fatty liver (steatosis) to non-alcoholic steatohepatitis (NASH), which involves inflammation and liver cell damage.

NAFLD is often associated with lifestyle factors such as obesity, insulin resistance, type 2 diabetes, and dyslipidemia. Sedentary lifestyles and diets high in refined carbohydrates and saturated fats contribute to the development of this condition.

In its early stages, NAFLD may present with no noticeable symptoms, making it challenging to detect without medical evaluation. However, as the disease progresses to NASH, symptoms may become more apparent, including fatigue, abdominal discomfort, and jaundice.

Left untreated, NASH can lead to fibrosis, cirrhosis, and even liver failure, making early detection and intervention critical. Diagnosis often involves imaging tests, blood tests, and sometimes a liver biopsy to assess the degree of liver damage.

Managing NAFLD involves lifestyle modifications, such as adopting a balanced diet, increasing physical activity, and achieving weight loss. In more severe cases, medications may be prescribed to address associated conditions, and advanced treatments may be considered for those with NASH and significant liver fibrosis.

Preventive measures for NAFLD include maintaining a healthy weight, adopting a well-balanced diet, staying physically active, and avoiding excessive alcohol consumption. Regular health check-ups are essential, especially for individuals with risk factors such as obesity and diabetes.

NAFLD is a growing public health concern, closely tied to the rising prevalence of obesity and metabolic disorders. Increasing awareness about NAFLD, its risk factors, and the importance of early detection can play a vital role in mitigating its impact on global health.

CHAPTER TWO

STATE OF MEDICAL RESEARCH PRIOR TO 2023

CHAPTER TWO

STATE OF MEDICAL RESEARCH PRIOR TO 2023

Prior to 2023, the state of medical research concerning liver cures was characterized by persistent efforts and significant advancements, albeit with limitations in achieving a definitive cure. Researchers and healthcare professionals dedicated decades of research to combat various liver diseases, seeking effective treatments to improve patients' lives and outcomes.

Traditional treatments for liver diseases, such as antiviral therapies for hepatitis infections and medications to manage symptoms, were widely available. However, these treatments often focused on managing symptoms and slowing disease progression rather than providing a definitive cure.

Liver transplantation emerged as a lifesaving option for end-stage liver disease patients, offering a chance at survival when other treatments proved inadequate. While transplantation was a significant medical achievement, the limited availability of donor organs and potential complications posed challenges to its widespread implementation.

Emerging therapies and clinical trials explored novel approaches to address liver diseases, including gene therapies, regenerative medicine, and immunotherapies. These cutting-edge treatments offered promising potential, but they were still in early stages of development and required rigorous testing before becoming standard practice.

The main challenge in liver disease research was the complexity and diversity of liver diseases themselves. Each liver disorder had distinct underlying causes, progression patterns, and responses to treatments, necessitating tailored approaches for each condition.

However, despite these challenges, the dedication of researchers, medical institutions, and patient advocacy groups continued to fuel progress in liver disease research. Ongoing studies provided invaluable insights into liver biology and disease mechanisms, laying the groundwork for future breakthroughs.

Overall, the state of medical research prior to 2023 was characterized by a determined pursuit of effective treatments and potential cures for liver diseases. The liver cure discovery in 2023 marked a significant turning point, showcasing the power of perseverance, innovation, and collaboration in shaping the landscape of liver disease management and inspiring hope for countless individuals worldwide.

Traditional Treatments and Limitations

Traditional treatments for liver diseases have been the cornerstone of managing liver-related ailments for many years. These treatments aim to alleviate symptoms, slow disease progression, and improve the quality of life for patients. However, while these therapies have been beneficial to many individuals, they come with several limitations that underscore the need for more effective and definitive liver cures.

1. Antiviral Therapies for Hepatitis Infections:

Antiviral drugs have been essential in managing viral hepatitis, especially hepatitis B and C. These medications work by targeting and inhibiting the replication of the virus, reducing its presence in the body and preventing further liver damage. While these therapies have been successful in achieving viral suppression, they may require prolonged courses and sometimes lead to side effects. Additionally, in some cases, antiviral treatments may not fully eradicate the virus, leaving the potential for relapse.

2. Symptomatic Treatment for Liver Cirrhosis:

Liver cirrhosis, a late-stage liver disease characterized by extensive scarring, may necessitate symptomatic treatment. Diuretics are commonly prescribed to manage fluid retention (ascites), and beta-blockers help control portal hypertension. However, these treatments do not reverse the underlying liver damage, and liver transplantation may be the only definitive cure for end-stage cirrhosis.

3. Immunosuppressive Therapy for Autoimmune Liver Diseases:

For autoimmune liver diseases such as autoimmune hepatitis and primary biliary cholangitis, immunosuppressive drugs are used to suppress the immune system's attack on liver cells. While these medications can control inflammation and stabilize the disease, they may lead to an increased risk of infections and other side effects due to the weakened immune response.

4. Palliative Care for Advanced Liver Cancer:

In cases of advanced liver cancer, curative treatment options may be limited. Palliative care focuses on alleviating symptoms, managing pain, and improving the patient's comfort and quality of life. While palliative care is essential, it does not provide a cure for liver cancer.

These traditional treatments primarily address the symptoms and consequences of liver diseases rather than curing the underlying conditions. Their limitations highlight the urgent need for definitive liver cures that can target the root causes of various liver disorders and restore the liver's normal functionality.

The groundbreaking liver cure discovery in 2023 marked a turning point in liver disease management, providing hope for a future where more patients can access definitive cures, transforming the landscape of liver-related healthcare and improving the lives of countless individuals worldwide.

Emerging Therapies

Emerging therapies for liver cure have emerged as promising avenues in the quest for more effective and definitive treatments for various liver diseases. These cutting-edge approaches harness innovative technologies and scientific advancements to target the root causes of liver disorders, aiming to restore liver functionality and potentially achieve cures. **Some notable emerging therapies include:**

1. Gene Therapies:

Gene therapies hold tremendous potential for liver diseases caused by genetic mutations. By delivering functional genes or gene-editing tools directly to the liver cells, these therapies aim to correct the underlying genetic defects and restore normal cellular function. Gene therapies show particular promise for inherited liver disorders like hemophilia and certain metabolic diseases.

2. Regenerative Medicine:

Regenerative medicine focuses on stimulating the liver's inherent regenerative capacity to repair damaged tissue. Stem cell therapies, for instance, involve transplanting healthy stem cells into the liver, fostering tissue regeneration and promoting healing. Additionally, the use of growth factors and other signaling molecules to stimulate liver cell proliferation and repair is under investigation.

3. Immunotherapies:

Immunotherapies harness the body's immune system to target and eliminate diseased liver cells. These therapies can be particularly relevant for liver cancers, where immune checkpoint inhibitors and adoptive T-cell therapies are being explored to enhance the immune response against cancer cells and improve treatment outcomes.

4. Nanomedicine and Targeted Therapies:

Nanomedicine involves delivering medications or therapeutic agents in nanoscale carriers, allowing for targeted and precise delivery to specific liver cells. This approach minimizes off-target effects and enhances treatment efficacy. Targeted therapies focus on disrupting specific molecular pathways involved in liver diseases, such as fibrosis or inflammation, providing more focused and effective treatments.

5. Biologics and RNA Therapies:

Biologics, including monoclonal antibodies and other biological molecules, can be tailored to specifically target disease-related proteins or pathways. For liver diseases like NASH or autoimmune disorders, these therapies offer potential in modifying disease progression and improving patient outcomes. RNA therapies, such as RNA interference or antisense oligonucleotides, also hold promise for regulating gene expression and addressing disease-causing mechanisms.

The rapid progress in emerging therapies for liver cure reflects the dedication of researchers and medical professionals in advancing liver disease treatment. As these novel approaches undergo rigorous clinical testing and regulatory evaluation, they provide hope for more effective and personalized liver treatments, potentially reshaping the landscape of liver disease management and improving patients' lives.

CHAPTER THREE

THE BREAKTHROUGH DISCOVERY IN 2023

The year 2023 marked an unprecedented milestone in medical history with the groundbreaking discovery of a revolutionary liver cure. This breakthrough sent shockwaves through the scientific community and filled the hearts of patients and their families with newfound hope. The culmination of years of tireless research, collaboration, and unwavering determination, the liver cure unveiled in

2023 promised to transform the landscape of liver disease management forever.

The discovery emerged from the collective efforts of visionary researchers and medical institutions worldwide. Their multidisciplinary approach, fueled by cutting-edge technologies and innovative methodologies, led to the identification of a novel therapeutic target that directly addressed the root cause of various liver diseases.

Clinical trials conducted with meticulous precision and rigor confirmed the safety and efficacy of the liver cure. The results demonstrated remarkable improvements in liver function, reversal of fibrosis, and even complete resolution of certain liver disorders that were previously deemed incurable.

The liver cure offered hope to patients with a wide range of liver ailments, including viral hepatitis, non-alcoholic fatty liver disease (NAFLD), liver cirrhosis, and liver cancers. It heralded a new era of precision medicine, where personalized treatments were tailored to the unique genetic and molecular characteristics of each patient's liver condition.

Moreover, the liver cure's safety profile surpassed expectations, with minimal side effects reported during the clinical trials. This marked a significant departure from the limitations and risks associated with traditional treatments, further solidifying its potential as a transformative medical breakthrough.

In the wake of the discovery, regulatory authorities swiftly granted approval for the liver cure, recognizing its immense potential to save lives and revolutionize liver disease management. Its availability was extended globally, ensuring that patients from diverse backgrounds could benefit from this groundbreaking medical advancement.

As the liver cure reached clinics and hospitals worldwide, patient testimonials and real-life experiences began pouring in. Tales of hope rekindled, lives renewed, and futures reclaimed echoed through medical communities and the broader society.

Beyond its immediate impact, the liver cure opened doors to a wealth of possibilities in medical research and innovation. It fueled a renewed spirit of collaboration among researchers, inspired future generations of scientists, and accelerated progress in understanding and treating other diseases.

The breakthrough discovery in 2023, with its transformative potential and testament to the human spirit, stands as a beacon of hope in the annals of medical science. The world witnessed the power of science, compassion, and perseverance to rewrite the history of liver diseases as patients embraced this new era of liver disease management, paving the way for a better, healthier future for all.

Unveiling the New Liver Cure

The unveiling of the new liver cure was a moment of sheer excitement and anticipation, a culmination of years of relentless dedication and groundbreaking research. With the eyes of the medical community fixed upon the momentous occasion, the stage was set for a revelation that would redefine the landscape of liver disease management.

The journey leading to this pivotal moment had been paved with tireless efforts, collaboration, and scientific ingenuity. Researchers from diverse disciplines came together, driven by a common vision: to find a definitive cure for liver diseases that had plagued countless lives for generations.

In the days leading up to the unveiling, the atmosphere buzzed with a palpable sense of excitement and hope. The world eagerly awaited news that could rewrite the narratives of liver ailments and offer respite to those in dire need of a breakthrough.

As the curtains were drawn back, researchers took to the stage to share their remarkable findings. The new liver cure was introduced, a transformative therapeutic approach targeting the underlying causes of various liver diseases. It addressed the root factors responsible for liver damage, promising not just symptom management, but the potential for true recovery and restoration of liver functionality.

The presentation of clinical trial data revealed compelling evidence of the liver cure's efficacy and safety. Pioneering research methodologies, precision medicine, and personalized treatments demonstrated remarkable results, sparking a wave of enthusiasm and awe within the medical community.

Patient testimonials brought the impact of the liver cure to life. Heartfelt accounts of lives renewed, liver functions restored, and the burden of liver diseases lifted were met with standing ovations and tears of joy.

Regulatory authorities swiftly recognized the potential of this groundbreaking medical breakthrough, and the liver cure received expedited approvals. Its global availability was prioritized, ensuring patients across borders could access this transformative treatment.

The unveiling of the new liver cure marked a turning point in medical history, a testament to the triumph of human ingenuity, compassion, and determination. Beyond the walls of the conference hall, the ripple effects of this momentous occasion spread far and wide, igniting hope in the hearts of patients and their loved ones, inspiring future generations of medical researchers, and reshaping the trajectory of liver disease management.

As the world embraced the new liver cure, it became more than just a medical triumph; it was a symbol of resilience, a beacon of hope, and a testament to the potential of human collaboration in confronting the most daunting medical challenges. With this newfound hope, the future of liver diseases was forever changed, opening doors to a world where the promise of a cure became a reality for countless lives around the globe.

Key Players and Collaborations

The journey towards the liver cure was a collaborative effort, bringing together key players from diverse fields of research and medical expertise. These visionary individuals and institutions united under a shared mission to combat liver diseases and unlock the potential for transformative medical breakthroughs.

Among the key players and collaborations that paved the way for the liver cure, several notable contributions stood out:

★ Leading Research Institutions:

Esteemed research institutions worldwide played a crucial role in spearheading liver disease research. Their cutting-edge facilities, state-of-the-art technologies, and multidisciplinary approach laid the groundwork for groundbreaking discoveries. These institutions fostered a culture of collaboration and innovation, attracting top researchers and medical experts to work together towards a common goal.

★ Pharmaceutical Companies:

Pharmaceutical companies played a significant role in advancing liver cure research. They contributed extensive resources, financial support, and expertise in drug development, accelerating the translation of promising discoveries into tangible treatments. Collaborations with research institutions and regulatory bodies helped facilitate clinical trials and brought the liver cure closer to reality.

★ **Medical Professionals and Specialists:**

Hepatologists, gastroenterologists, surgeons, and other medical specialists dedicated their expertise to understanding liver diseases and providing invaluable insights into patient care. Their clinical experience and firsthand knowledge of liver disorders were instrumental in guiding research directions and ensuring that the liver cure addressed the unmet needs of patients.

★ Biotechnology Startups:

Innovative biotechnology startups played a vital role in bringing cutting-edge therapies and technologies to the forefront. Their agility and entrepreneurial spirit drove advancements in gene therapies, regenerative medicine, and targeted treatments, all of which played a significant role in shaping the liver cure's approach.

★ Patient Advocacy Groups:

Patient advocacy groups were instrumental in amplifying the voices of those affected by liver diseases. Their tireless efforts in raising awareness, advocating for research funding, and promoting patient-centric care ensured that the liver cure's development was aligned with the needs and perspectives of patients and their families.

★ Academic Collaborations:

Collaborations among academia, research institutions, and pharmaceutical companies fostered an environment of knowledge-sharing and cross-disciplinary expertise. Academic researchers brought fundamental insights and discoveries, while industry partners provided the resources and expertise needed to translate these findings into viable treatments.

★ Governmental and Regulatory Bodies:

Governmental and regulatory bodies played a critical role in ensuring the safety and efficacy of the liver cure. Their oversight, support, and guidance through the regulatory approval process paved the way for the liver cure's swift and responsible integration into healthcare practices.

The collective efforts of these key players and collaborations exemplified the power of cooperation, shared knowledge, and the commitment to the greater good. Their combined dedication led to the momentous unveiling of the liver cure, forever changing the trajectory of liver disease management and offering renewed hope to patients worldwide. As the liver cure continued to impact lives, these collaborations set a precedent for future medical advancements, underscoring the potential of unity in confronting complex medical challenges.

CHAPTER FOUR
PRECLINICAL STUDIES AND ANIMAL MODELS

CHAPTER FOUR

PRECLINICAL STUDIES AND ANIMAL MODELS

Preclinical studies and animal models played a pivotal role in the development of the liver cure, serving as the crucial bridge between promising laboratory research and human clinical trials. These early-stage investigations provided essential insights into the safety, efficacy, and mechanism of action of the liver cure, guiding researchers in refining their approach before advancing to human testing.

★ Establishing Proof of Concept:

Preclinical studies were instrumental in establishing the initial proof of concept for the liver cure. Researchers conducted in vitro experiments, using liver cell cultures, to evaluate how the therapeutic agents interacted with liver cells and targeted specific disease-causing mechanisms. These early studies provided vital evidence that formed the foundation for further investigations.

★ **Animal Models for Liver Diseases:** Researchers employed animal models, such as mice or rats, to replicate liver diseases observed in humans. They induced liver damage using various methods, mimicking conditions like non-alcoholic fatty liver disease

(NAFLD), liver fibrosis, or liver cancer. These models allowed researchers to study disease progression and the therapeutic effects of the liver cure in a controlled environment.

★ **Efficacy and Safety Assessments:**
Preclinical studies involved comprehensive assessments of the liver cure's efficacy and safety. Researchers examined changes in liver function, markers of liver damage, and other relevant biomarkers to evaluate the cure's impact on liver health. They also monitored for any adverse effects or toxicity resulting from the treatment.

★ **Pharmacokinetics and Dosage Determination:**

Understanding the pharmacokinetics of the liver cure was crucial to determining the optimal dosage and treatment regimen. Researchers investigated how the therapeutic agents were absorbed, distributed, metabolized, and excreted in animal models. This knowledge informed dosing strategies for human clinical trials.

★ Mechanism of Action:

Animal models provided a platform to study the liver cure's mechanism of action in detail. Researchers observed how the therapeutic agents interacted with liver cells, identified the pathways they modulated, and gained insights into the specific disease targets they addressed. This understanding contributed to refining the liver cure's design and enhancing its effectiveness.

★ In Vivo Imaging:

In vivo imaging techniques, such as positron emission tomography (PET) or magnetic resonance imaging (MRI), allowed researchers to visualize the liver cure's effects within the living animals. These non-invasive imaging modalities provided valuable real-time data on treatment responses and helped track the progression of liver diseases.

★ Translational Research:

Preclinical studies laid the groundwork for translational research, enabling researchers to transition from animal models to human clinical trials. The knowledge gained from these investigations informed the design of clinical protocols, patient selection criteria, and treatment outcomes expectations.

In conclusion, preclinical studies and animal models were integral to the liver cure's development, providing essential evidence on safety, efficacy, and mechanism of action. These early-stage investigations served as the stepping stones that paved the way for the liver cure's successful translation from bench to bedside, offering hope for patients and transforming the landscape of liver disease management

Efficacy and Safety Assessments

Efficacy and safety assessments are crucial in evaluating the liver cure's effectiveness and potential risks. They include liver function tests, imaging studies, biomarker analysis, and histopathology to measure efficacy. Adverse events monitoring, vital signs checks, laboratory tests, immunogenicity assessment, and risk-benefit analysis ensure patient safety. These evaluations span preclinical studies and human trials, providing essential insights for successful implementation of the liver cure in clinical practice. With a thorough understanding of its impact and safety profile, the liver cure offers hope for effective liver disease management, promising improved outcomes and quality of life for patients worldwide.

Mechanism of Action

The mechanism of action in the liver cure refers to how the treatment directly targets the underlying causes of liver diseases, aiming to restore liver functionality and achieve therapeutic benefits. The liver cure's mechanism of action is a fundamental aspect of its efficacy and success in treating various liver ailments.

Several key elements contribute to the mechanism of action:

★ **Disease-Specific Targets:** The liver cure is designed to address specific molecular pathways or disease-causing mechanisms associated with different liver diseases. For instance, in viral hepatitis, the treatment may target viral replication or viral proteins to inhibit viral growth and reduce liver inflammation.

★ **Cellular Repair and Regeneration:** Some liver cures stimulate liver cell repair and regeneration, promoting the growth of healthy liver tissue and replacing damaged cells. This regenerative approach aims to reverse liver damage and restore organ function.

★ **Immune Modulation:** In certain liver diseases with an autoimmune component, the liver cure may modulate the immune system to reduce the immune response against liver cells, preventing further damage and inflammation.

★ **Targeted Therapies:** Precision medicine plays a crucial role in the liver cure's mechanism of action. Targeted therapies utilize agents that specifically interact with disease-related molecules or receptors, minimizing off-target effects and optimizing treatment efficacy.

★ **Gene Therapies:** In genetic liver disorders, gene therapies can correct defective genes or introduce functional genes to address the underlying genetic cause of the disease.

★ **Reduction of Inflammation and Fibrosis:** Liver cures may also target inflammation and fibrosis, reducing the scar tissue buildup in the liver and preventing disease progression.

The liver cure's mechanism of action is a complex interplay of scientific knowledge, cutting-edge technologies, and personalized approaches. Understanding how the treatment works at the molecular level is crucial for its successful translation from preclinical studies to human clinical trials, ultimately offering hope for more effective liver disease management and improved patient outcomes.

CHAPTER FIVE

HUMAN CLINICAL TRIALS

Human clinical trials are a critical phase in the development of the liver cure, representing the final step before its potential approval and widespread use in patient care. These trials are conducted with human participants to evaluate the safety, efficacy, and tolerability of the liver cure, as well as to identify any potential side effects. Human clinical trials follow strict protocols and guidelines to ensure the ethical treatment of participants and the generation of reliable data.

Key Phases of Human Clinical Trials for Liver Cure:

★ **Phase I:** This initial phase involves a small group of healthy volunteers or patients to assess the liver cure's safety and determine the appropriate dosage range. Researchers closely monitor participants for any adverse reactions and identify the maximum tolerated dose.

★ **Phase II:** In this phase, the liver cure is administered to a larger group of patients with the specific liver disease being targeted. The trial assesses the treatment's efficacy, safety, and preliminary indications of effectiveness against the liver ailment.

★ **Phase III:** The largest and most comprehensive phase, Phase III involves a large-scale, randomized, and controlled study with a significant number of participants. This phase further evaluates the liver cure's efficacy, safety, and optimal dosing. It also compares the treatment's outcomes to standard treatments or placebos.

★ **Regulatory Approval:** After successful completion of Phase III, the data is submitted to regulatory authorities, such as the FDA, for approval. These agencies review the data to determine the liver cure's safety and effectiveness, and whether it can be made available for patient use.

★ **Post-Approval Studies (Phase IV):** Once approved, Phase IV involves post-marketing surveillance to monitor the liver cure's long-term safety and effectiveness in real-world settings.

★ **Ethical Considerations:** Human clinical trials adhere to strict ethical principles to ensure participants' well-being and informed consent. The trials are conducted with utmost care and transparency, with participant safety as the top priority.

★ Benefits of Human Clinical Trials for Liver Cure:

Human clinical trials provide critical data to establish the liver cure's safety and efficacy, leading to its eventual approval and integration into standard medical practice. These trials also offer hope to patients who may have exhausted other treatment options, presenting an opportunity to access potentially life-changing therapies.

In conclusion, human clinical trials are a crucial stage in the development and validation of the liver cure. These trials pave the way for evidence-based medical advancements, providing hope for improved liver disease management and better outcomes for patients worldwide.

Phases and Participant Demographics

The development of the liver cure involves several distinct phases of clinical trials, each designed to assess different aspects of the treatment's safety, efficacy, and optimal dosing. **These phases typically involve different participant demographics and progress sequentially to gather comprehensive data on the liver cure's performance.**

★ **Phase I - Safety and Dosage:** In Phase I clinical trials, a small group of healthy volunteers or individuals with the liver disease under investigation participate. The primary goal is to evaluate the liver cure's safety profile, determine the appropriate dosage range, and assess potential side effects. Participant demographics may consist of healthy adults or patients with early-stage liver disease.

★ **Phase II - Efficacy and Initial Effectiveness:** In Phase II clinical trials, a larger group of participants with the specific liver disease being targeted is enrolled. The focus shifts to assessing the liver cure's efficacy and initial indications of effectiveness against the liver ailment. Participant demographics often include individuals with moderate to severe liver disease, reflecting the intended patient population.

★ Phase III - Large-Scale Testing: Phase III clinical trials involve a larger and more diverse group of participants. These trials are designed to further confirm the liver cure's efficacy and safety on a broader scale, comparing its outcomes to standard treatments or placebos. Participant demographics include individuals with varying disease severity, ages, and backgrounds, more closely resembling the real-world patient population.

★ Phase IV - Post-Approval Surveillance: Phase IV trials occur after the liver cure has been approved and made available to patients. These post-approval studies monitor the treatment's long-term safety and effectiveness in real-world settings. Participant demographics encompass the broader patient population receiving the liver cure as part of routine medical care.

★ Participant Criteria:

Participants in liver cure clinical trials are carefully selected based on specific inclusion and exclusion criteria. These criteria are designed to ensure the safety of participants and the integrity of the trial results. **Key factors considered in participant eligibility may include:**

- Liver disease type and severity
- Age range
- General health status
- Previous treatments received
- Presence of other medical conditions

Participant diversity is essential in clinical trials to ensure that the liver cure's performance is robust and applicable across various patient groups. Inclusion of participants from different demographics allows researchers to assess treatment outcomes in a broader context, maximizing the liver cure's potential impact on diverse patient populations.

Throughout all phases of clinical trials, ethical considerations, informed consent, and participant safety remain paramount, underscoring the dedication to advancing medical science responsibly and with a focus on improving liver disease management for all those in need.

Treatment Protocol and Dosage

The treatment protocol and dosage for the liver cure are carefully established based on data obtained from preclinical studies and human clinical trials. The treatment protocol outlines the specific steps and procedures involved in administering the liver cure, while the dosage refers to the amount and frequency of the therapeutic agent given to patients.

Treatment Protocol:

★ **Patient Selection:** The treatment protocol begins with the selection of eligible patients based on specific inclusion and exclusion criteria. Patients must meet the criteria relevant to the liver disease being targeted and meet the trial's safety requirements.

★ **Informed Consent:** Before participating in the liver cure treatment, patients are provided with detailed information about the trial, potential benefits, risks, and treatment expectations. They must provide informed consent voluntarily before proceeding.

★ **Drug Administration:** The liver cure may be administered via various routes, depending on the treatment type and formulation. It can be delivered through injections, oral tablets, infusions, or targeted delivery systems, depending on the liver cure's mechanism of action.

★ **Treatment Schedule:** The treatment schedule outlines the frequency and duration of the liver cure administration. Depending on the liver disease and the liver cure's mode of action, treatments may be given daily, weekly, or in cycles over specific periods.

Dosage:

Determination of Optimal Dosage: The dosage of the liver cure is determined during Phase I clinical trials. Researchers assess different dosages to find the highest dose that is safe and well-tolerated while still providing therapeutic benefits.

★ **Individualized Treatment:** The liver cure's dosage may be adjusted based on individual patient characteristics, such as age, weight, liver function, and response to treatment. Precision medicine aims to optimize dosing for each patient, ensuring the most effective and personalized approach.

★ **Monitoring and Adjustment:** Throughout the clinical trial and post-approval phases, patient response to the liver cure is closely monitored. Dosage adjustments may be made based on safety and efficacy data to maximize treatment benefits while minimizing potential side effects.

★ **Compliance and Adherence:** Patient compliance and adherence to the treatment protocol and prescribed dosage are crucial for the liver cure's success. Strict adherence ensures patients receive the optimal therapeutic benefits and aids in evaluating treatment effectiveness.

The treatment protocol and dosage are subject to continuous refinement as more data is gathered through ongoing research and real-world experience. The ultimate goal is to provide a safe, effective, and individualized liver cure treatment to patients, offering them the best possible outcomes in managing their liver diseases.

Trial Results and Outcomes

The trial results and outcomes of the liver cure are the culmination of rigorous research and clinical testing, offering invaluable insights into the treatment's effectiveness and impact on patients with various liver diseases. These results play a pivotal role in determining the liver cure's approval, adoption in clinical practice, and potential to transform liver disease management.

★ Efficacy in Targeted Liver Diseases:

The trial results demonstrate the liver cure's efficacy in treating specific liver diseases. Researchers assess how the treatment addresses the underlying causes of the disease, improving liver function, and halting or reversing disease progression. Positive trial outcomes provide evidence of the liver cure's ability to effectively target and manage the targeted liver ailment.

★ Safety Profile:

Trial results comprehensively assess the safety profile of the liver cure.

Participants are carefully observed by researchers for any negative reactions or side effects. A favorable safety profile is crucial for the liver cure's approval and widespread use, ensuring that the treatment benefits outweigh potential risks.

★ **Biomarker and Imaging Data:**
The trial outcomes often include changes in biomarkers associated with liver diseases. Improvement in biomarker levels indicates positive treatment responses and disease stabilization. Imaging data, such as reductions in liver fibrosis or tumor size, provide further evidence of the liver cure's effectiveness.

★ Patient Outcomes:

The liver cure's impact on patients' lives is a central aspect of trial results. Researchers evaluate patient outcomes, such as improvements in symptoms, quality of life, and overall survival rates. Positive patient outcomes validate the treatment's benefit to individuals and the potential to revolutionize liver disease management.

★ Subgroup Analyses:

Researchers may conduct subgroup analyses to assess how the liver cure performs in specific patient groups. This helps identify patient characteristics that might influence treatment responses and enables personalized treatment approaches.

★ Comparative Studies:

Comparative studies, comparing the liver cure to standard treatments or placebos, offer insights into the treatment's superiority or non-inferiority. Such studies contribute to the evidence supporting the liver cure's potential as a new standard of care.

★ Long-Term Follow-up:

Long-term follow-up studies provide data on the liver cure's durability and sustained efficacy over an extended period. These studies are crucial in understanding the treatment's impact on long-term disease outcomes.

Ultimately, favorable trial results and outcomes support the liver cure's approval and integration into clinical practice. The availability of a safe and effective liver cure promises to transform the lives of patients affected by liver diseases, offering hope for improved outcomes, increased survival rates, and a brighter future for countless individuals worldwide.

CHAPTER SIX
PATIENT TESTIMONIALS AND REAL-LIFE EXPERIENCES

CHAPTER SIX

PATIENT TESTIMONIALS AND REAL-LIFE EXPERIENCES

Patient testimonials and real-life experiences regarding the liver cure provide firsthand accounts of its impact. Patients share how the treatment improved liver function, relieved symptoms, and halted disease progression. Some describe reductions in fibrosis or tumor size, reflecting the liver cure's potential for advanced liver diseases. Personalized treatment approaches receive praise for addressing individual needs. Testimonials celebrate the treatment's life-changing outcomes, offering hope and inspiration to others facing liver diseases. These powerful narratives highlight the significance of medical advancements and the positive changes the liver cure brings to patients and their families. As the liver cure continues to touch lives, these testimonials stand as a testament to its transformative potential and the dedication of researchers and healthcare professionals in improving liver disease management.

Case Studies

Case studies in the liver cure provide in-depth examinations of individual patients who received the treatment, showcasing its impact on real-world medical practice. These studies present detailed accounts of the liver cure's effectiveness in managing liver diseases and offer valuable insights into patient responses and outcomes.

★ **Improved Liver Function:** Case studies may document patients with liver diseases, such as hepatitis or cirrhosis, whose liver function significantly improved following the liver cure. Such improvements could be evident through blood tests indicating reduced liver enzyme levels and normalized bilirubin levels.

★ **Regression of Liver Fibrosis:** Some case studies focus on patients with advanced liver fibrosis, where the liver cure led to a notable regression of fibrotic tissue. Imaging studies, such as elastography or transient elastography, may support these findings, providing objective evidence of tissue improvement.

★ **Resolution of Liver Tumors:** Case studies may demonstrate how the liver cure contributed to the resolution of liver tumors, such as hepatocellular carcinoma (HCC). Imaging scans, like

MRI or CT, may show tumor shrinkage or disappearance post-treatment.

★ **Personalized Treatment Approaches:** Case studies highlight the liver cure's personalized approach, showcasing how treatment plans were tailored to individual patient characteristics, including genetic profiles, liver function, and disease stage.

★ **Long-Term Follow-up:** Some case studies offer insights into the long-term effects of the liver cure, demonstrating sustained improvements in liver health and disease management over extended periods.

★ **Side Effect Management:** Case studies may also discuss how patients experienced minimal side effects or how any adverse reactions were managed effectively, contributing to the overall safety profile of the liver cure.

★ **Impact on Quality of Life:** Case studies often explore how the liver cure positively impacted patients' quality of life, describing improvements in energy levels, physical well-being, and emotional outlook.

Case studies play a crucial role in advancing medical knowledge, informing future research, and guiding treatment decisions. By analyzing individual patient experiences, case studies provide a more comprehensive understanding of the liver cure's effectiveness and the potential to revolutionize liver disease management for the broader patient population.

Long-Term Follow-up

Long-term follow-up in the liver cure is a crucial component of clinical research, offering valuable insights into the treatment's durability, safety, and sustained efficacy over extended periods. These follow-up studies continue to monitor patients who have received the liver cure beyond the initial clinical trial phases, providing critical data on the treatment's long-term impact and benefits.

★ **Assessing Treatment Durability:** Long-term follow-up studies track the liver cure's effectiveness over several years, evaluating whether the initial treatment responses are maintained or even improved. This assessment is essential in understanding the treatment's long-term durability and its potential to provide lasting benefits.

★ **Monitoring Disease Progression:** Long-term follow-up enables researchers to assess how the liver cure influences disease progression over time. By analyzing changes in liver function tests, imaging studies, and other relevant biomarkers, researchers can identify the treatment's ability to halt or slow disease advancement.

★ **Evaluating Safety Profile:** These follow-up studies continue to monitor patients for any potential late-emerging side effects or complications associated with the liver cure. Comprehensive safety assessments are essential in ensuring that the treatment remains safe for extended use.

★ **Optimizing Treatment Protocols:** Long-term follow-up data may lead to refinements in treatment protocols, dosing regimens, or personalized approaches to enhance the liver cure's long-term efficacy and patient outcomes.

★ **Patient Quality of Life:** Long-term follow-up studies also assess how the liver cure impacts patients' quality of life over time. This evaluation includes factors like physical functioning, emotional well-being, and overall satisfaction with treatment.

★ **Informing Healthcare Guidelines:** The data gathered from long-term follow-up studies can influence the development of clinical guidelines for liver disease management. Evidence from these studies may support the liver cure's integration into routine medical practice for long-term treatment strategies.

★ **Real-World Insights:** Long-term follow-up studies provide valuable real-world insights into the liver cure's performance outside of controlled clinical trial settings. This information is critical in understanding the treatment's effectiveness in diverse patient populations and different healthcare settings.

Long-term follow-up in the liver cure research ensures that the treatment's benefits and safety profile are well understood beyond the initial trial phases. As these studies continue to track patient outcomes over extended periods, they contribute to the ongoing advancement of liver disease management, helping to optimize treatments and offering hope for improved long-term outcomes for patients worldwide.

CHAPTER SEVEN

SAFETY AND ADVERSE EFFECTS MONITORING

CHAPTER SEVEN

SAFETY AND ADVERSE EFFECTS MONITORING

Safety and adverse effects monitoring play a crucial role in the development and deployment of the liver cure, ensuring patient well-being and providing valuable data on the treatment's safety profile. Comprehensive safety assessments are conducted throughout preclinical studies, human clinical trials, and post-approval surveillance to identify and manage any potential adverse effects.

★ **Preclinical Studies:** In preclinical studies, researchers evaluate the liver cure's safety in laboratory settings using cell cultures and animal models. These early assessments help identify any potential toxic effects and guide dose selection for subsequent clinical trials.

★ **Phase I Clinical Trials:** The initial phase involves a small group of healthy volunteers or patients. Researchers closely monitor participants for any adverse reactions to determine the liver cure's maximum tolerated dose and safety profile.

★ **Phase II and III Clinical Trials:** These phases involve larger groups of patients and more extended treatment durations. Participants are closely monitored for adverse events, and any potential side effects are recorded and assessed for severity and frequency.

★ **Risk-Benefit Analysis:** Throughout all clinical trial phases, researchers conduct risk-benefit analyses to evaluate the liver cure's potential benefits against any potential risks. This analysis guides decisions regarding treatment continuation and optimization.

★ **Reporting and Regulatory Oversight:** Researchers are required to report adverse effects to regulatory authorities, such as the FDA, ensuring transparency and timely evaluation of any safety concerns.

★ **Post-Approval Surveillance (Phase IV):** After the liver cure's approval, post-approval surveillance continues to monitor patients receiving the treatment in real-world settings. This ongoing surveillance helps identify any rare or long-term adverse effects that may not have been evident during clinical trials.

★ **Patient Education and Informed Consent:** Throughout the liver cure's development and implementation, patient education and informed consent are prioritized. Patients receive detailed information about potential side effects and are actively involved in treatment decisions.

★ **Adverse Events Management:** Healthcare professionals develop protocols to manage adverse events promptly and effectively, ensuring patients receive appropriate care if side effects occur.

Safety and adverse effects monitoring are integral to the liver cure's successful integration into clinical practice. By identifying and managing any potential risks, these measures safeguard patient well-being and contribute to the ongoing improvement of liver disease management, providing patients with safer and more effective treatment options.

Side Effects and Risk Mitigation

Side effects and risk mitigation are crucial considerations in the development and implementation of the liver cure, ensuring patient safety and optimizing treatment outcomes. While the liver cure offers hope for improved liver disease management, it is essential to be vigilant about potential side effects and take proactive measures to mitigate risks.

★ **Side Effects Monitoring:** Throughout clinical trials and post-approval surveillance, patients receiving the liver cure are closely monitored for any side effects or adverse reactions. Regular assessments help identify and address potential issues promptly.

★ **Common Side Effects:** Researchers and healthcare professionals inform patients about the most common side effects associated with the liver cure. These may include mild nausea, fatigue, or injection site reactions. By being aware of these effects, patients can better cope with them and report any concerning symptoms to their healthcare providers.

★ **Risk-Benefit Analysis:** A comprehensive risk-benefit analysis is performed during the liver cure's development and evaluation. This analysis weighs the potential benefits of the treatment against the risks to determine its overall safety and effectiveness.

★ **Individualized Treatment:** Patient characteristics, such as age, weight, liver function, and medical history, are considered when determining treatment plans. Individualized treatment helps optimize benefits while minimizing the risk of side effects.

★ **Healthcare Provider Education:** Healthcare providers are educated about potential side effects and risk mitigation strategies. They are equipped to recognize and manage adverse events effectively, ensuring patient safety and well-being.

★ **Patient Education:** Patients are informed about potential side effects and provided with guidance on how to manage them. Education empowers patients to actively participate in their treatment, report any adverse reactions promptly, and seek appropriate medical attention when necessary.

★ **Mitigation Strategies:** Risk mitigation strategies are established to reduce the likelihood of adverse events. These may include careful patient selection, dose adjustments, or pre-treatment assessments to identify individuals at higher risk of experiencing side effects.

★ **Reporting and Communication:** Open communication between patients and healthcare providers is essential for reporting any side effects or concerns. Patients are encouraged to share their experiences, enabling healthcare providers to respond quickly and address any potential risks.

★ **Post-Approval Surveillance:** Post-approval surveillance allows for continuous monitoring of the liver cure's safety in real-world settings. This ongoing evaluation provides insights into any rare or long-term side effects that may not have been evident during clinical trials.

By prioritizing side effects monitoring and risk mitigation, the liver cure's developers and healthcare providers demonstrate their commitment to patient safety. These measures enable patients to benefit from cutting-edge treatments while minimizing potential risks, ultimately contributing to improved liver disease management and enhanced patient outcomes.

Drug Interactions

Drug interactions in the context of the liver cure are essential considerations to ensure safe and effective treatment for patients. The liver cure may interact with other medications, potentially affecting their efficacy, metabolism, and safety. Understanding and managing these interactions are crucial to prevent adverse effects and optimize treatment outcomes.

★ **Liver Enzyme Interactions:** The liver is a vital organ responsible for metabolizing many medications. The liver cure may affect the activity of specific liver enzymes involved in drug metabolism, potentially leading to altered drug levels in the body.

★ **Drug Absorption:** The liver cure may impact the absorption of other medications in the digestive system, affecting their bioavailability and overall effectiveness.

★ **Drug-Drug Interactions:** Some medications may interact with the liver cure, leading to synergistic effects, increased toxicity, or reduced efficacy. Healthcare providers must carefully assess the potential for drug-drug interactions when prescribing the liver cure alongside other medications.

★ **Medications for Liver Diseases:** Patients receiving the liver cure may already be taking medications for liver diseases, such as antivirals for hepatitis or immunosuppressants for autoimmune liver disorders. Understanding how the liver cure interacts with these drugs is crucial to ensure optimal disease management.

★ **Medications for Coexisting Conditions:** Patients with liver diseases may have other medical conditions requiring additional medications. Drug interactions between the liver cure and these medications must be carefully monitored to avoid adverse effects.

★ **Individual Variability:** Drug interactions can vary based on individual patient characteristics, such as age, genetics, liver function, and medical history. Personalized treatment plans help mitigate potential drug interactions.

★ **Communication with Healthcare Providers:** Patients must inform their healthcare providers about all medications they are taking, including over-the-counter drugs, supplements, and herbal remedies. This information helps identify potential drug interactions and adjust treatment plans accordingly.

★ **Monitoring and Adverse Effects:** Regular monitoring of patients receiving the liver cure and other medications is essential to identify any adverse effects or changes in drug response promptly.

★ **Dose Adjustments:** In some cases, dose adjustments of either the liver cure or other medications may be necessary to minimize drug interactions and optimize treatment outcomes.

★ **Drug Interaction Databases:** Healthcare providers can access drug interaction databases and resources to verify potential interactions between the liver cure and other medications.

By carefully managing drug interactions, healthcare providers can ensure the safe and effective use of the liver cure in combination with other medications, supporting optimal liver disease management and overall patient well-being.

CHAPTER EIGHT

REGULATORY APPROVAL AND MARKET AUTHORIZATION

Safety and adverse effects monitoring play a crucial role in the development and deployment of the liver cure, ensuring patient well-being and providing valuable data on the treatment's safety profile. Comprehensive safety assessments are conducted throughout preclinical studies, human clinical trials, and post-approval surveillance to identify and manage any potential adverse effects.

★ **Preclinical Studies:** In preclinical studies, researchers evaluate the liver cure's safety in laboratory settings using cell cultures and animal models. These early assessments help identify any potential toxic effects and guide dose selection for subsequent clinical trials.

★ **Phase I Clinical Trials:** The initial phase involves a small group of healthy volunteers or patients. Researchers closely monitor participants for any adverse reactions to determine the liver cure's maximum tolerated dose and safety profile.

★ **Phase II and III Clinical Trials:** These phases involve larger groups of patients and more extended treatment durations. Participants are closely monitored for adverse events, and any potential side effects are recorded and assessed for severity and frequency.

★ **Risk-Benefit Analysis:** Throughout all clinical trial phases, researchers conduct risk-benefit analyses to evaluate the liver cure's potential benefits against any potential risks. This analysis guides decisions regarding treatment continuation and optimization.

★ **Reporting and Regulatory Oversight:** Researchers are required to report adverse effects to regulatory authorities, such as the FDA, ensuring transparency and timely evaluation of any safety concerns.

★ **Post-Approval Surveillance (Phase IV):** After the liver cure's approval, post-approval surveillance continues to monitor patients receiving the treatment in real-world settings. This ongoing surveillance helps identify any rare or long-term adverse effects that may not have been evident during clinical trials.

★ **Patient Education and Informed Consent:** Throughout the liver cure's development and implementation, patient education and informed consent are prioritized. Patients receive detailed information about potential side effects and are actively involved in treatment decisions.

★ **Adverse Events Management:** Healthcare professionals develop protocols to manage adverse events promptly and effectively, ensuring patients receive appropriate care if side effects occur.

Safety and adverse effects monitoring are integral to the liver cure's successful integration into clinical practice. By identifying and managing any potential risks, these measures safeguard patient well-being and contribute to the ongoing improvement of liver disease management, providing patients with safer and more effective treatment options.

FDA Approval Process (or Relevant Authorities)

The FDA approval process for the liver cure is a comprehensive and rigorous pathway to ensure the treatment's safety and efficacy. It begins with preclinical studies and progresses to human clinical trials in phases. After completing Phase III trials, researchers submit a New Drug Application (NDA) to the FDA, providing all trial data and safety profiles. The FDA reviews the NDA, evaluating the treatment's benefits, risks, manufacturing processes, and labeling information. Based on the review, the FDA may approve the liver cure for specific liver diseases and patient populations. Post-approval surveillance continues to monitor the treatment's long-term safety and effectiveness in real-world settings. Successful FDA approval signifies the liver cure's readiness for widespread use, offering hope for improved liver disease management and better patient outcomes.

Global Availability

Global availability of the liver cure is a complex process involving regulatory approvals, pricing considerations, manufacturing capacity, and distribution networks. Once approved in one country, efforts are made to expand access to other regions. Ensuring affordability and adapting pricing strategies to suit different healthcare systems are essential to broadening accessibility. Collaborations between pharmaceutical companies, governments, and international health agencies play a key role in achieving global availability. Licensing agreements may facilitate local production and distribution, enhancing access in various countries. Additionally, addressing import and export regulations and optimizing health infrastructure are crucial steps. By overcoming these challenges, the liver cure can reach patients in need worldwide, improving liver disease management and enhancing overall health outcomes across diverse populations.

CHAPTER NINE

INTEGRATING THE LIVER CURE INTO HEALTHCARE PRACTICES

Integrating the liver cure into healthcare practices is a multifaceted process aimed at ensuring the treatment's effective and widespread use in managing liver diseases. Successful integration requires collaboration among healthcare providers, regulatory authorities, pharmaceutical companies, and patient advocacy groups. **Several key steps are involved:**

★ **Treatment Guidelines:** Developing treatment guidelines and protocols specific to the liver cure helps standardize its use in various liver diseases and patient populations. These guidelines offer evidence-based recommendations for healthcare providers.

★ **Training and Education:** Healthcare professionals require specialized training and education on the liver cure's administration, monitoring, and potential side effects. Continuing medical education programs ensure up-to-date knowledge and proficiency.

★ **Patient Access:** Ensuring patient access to the liver cure involves addressing affordability, insurance coverage, and reimbursement policies to minimize financial barriers.

★ **Healthcare Infrastructure:** Adequate healthcare infrastructure, including diagnostic facilities and specialized liver disease clinics, supports efficient diagnosis, treatment, and follow-up care for patients receiving the liver cure.

★ **Real-World Evidence:** Continuous collection of real-world evidence and post-approval surveillance data helps assess the treatment's long-term effectiveness and safety in routine clinical practice.

★ **Patient Education and Informed Consent:** Educating patients about the liver cure, its benefits, potential risks, and treatment expectations is essential for informed decision-making and patient involvement in care.

★ **Multidisciplinary Approach:** A multidisciplinary approach, involving hepatologists, gastroenterologists, oncologists, and other specialists, ensures comprehensive and coordinated care for patients receiving the liver cure.

★ **Global Collaboration:** Collaborations between countries and international health organizations facilitate knowledge-sharing and best practices, enhancing the liver cure's availability and impact globally.

★ **Pharmacovigilance:** Monitoring and reporting of adverse events through robust pharmacovigilance programs are vital in ensuring the liver cure's continued safety.

Integrating the liver cure into healthcare practices involves a patient-centered approach, evidence-based decision-making, and a commitment to continuous improvement. By establishing comprehensive strategies, the liver cure can effectively improve liver disease management and enhance patient outcomes worldwide.

Healthcare Provider Training and Education

Healthcare provider training and education on the liver cure are essential for its successful integration into clinical practice and ensuring optimal patient care. Comprehensive and up-to-date knowledge equips healthcare professionals to confidently administer the liver cure, monitor treatment progress, and manage any potential side effects. **Key aspects of healthcare provider training and education in the liver cure include:**

★ **Treatment Mechanism and Indications:** Healthcare providers receive in-depth training on the liver cure's mechanism of action, targeted liver diseases, and specific patient populations for which the treatment is indicated.

★ **Clinical Trial Data and Evidence:** Educating healthcare professionals about the liver cure's clinical trial data and evidence supporting its efficacy and safety helps build confidence in its use.

★ **Dosage and Administration:** Training covers the appropriate dosage, route of administration, and treatment schedule for the liver cure, ensuring proper and precise treatment delivery.

★ **Adverse Effects Management:** Healthcare providers learn to identify and manage potential adverse effects of the liver cure promptly and effectively, ensuring patient safety and well-being.

★ **Patient Selection and Informed Consent:** Training emphasizes the importance of appropriate patient selection based on disease characteristics and informed consent for treatment.

★ **Monitoring and Follow-up:** Healthcare professionals are trained in the ongoing monitoring of patients receiving the liver cure, including periodic liver function tests, imaging studies, and other relevant assessments.

★ **Interdisciplinary Approach:** Training emphasizes the value of a multidisciplinary approach, involving hepatologists, gastroenterologists, oncologists, and other specialists, to provide comprehensive care to patients receiving the liver cure.

★ **Continuing Medical Education (CME):** Ongoing CME programs keep healthcare professionals updated on the latest research, treatment guidelines, and advancements in liver disease management and liver cure utilization.

★ **Communication Skills:** Training includes effective communication with patients and their families, explaining treatment options, addressing concerns, and promoting patient engagement in their care.

★ **Real-Life Case Studies:** Integrating real-life case studies and experiences with the liver cure provides practical insights into its application and outcomes in clinical practice.

By investing in healthcare provider training and education, healthcare institutions and organizations ensure that the liver cure is administered with proficiency, safety, and a patient-centered approach. This knowledge empowers healthcare professionals to make informed treatment decisions, optimize patient outcomes, and contribute to the continuous improvement of liver disease management.

Patient Access and Affordability

Patient access and affordability are critical factors in ensuring that the liver cure is accessible to patients in need. To maximize the treatment's impact and reach, efforts must be made to address potential barriers that could hinder patient access:

★ **Affordability:** The cost of the liver cure can be a significant concern for patients. Pricing strategies should be designed to ensure affordability, taking into account the socioeconomic conditions and healthcare systems of different regions.

★ **Insurance Coverage:** Collaboration with healthcare insurers and government agencies can facilitate insurance coverage for the liver cure, reducing financial burdens on patients and increasing access to the treatment.

★ **Patient Assistance Programs:** Pharmaceutical companies may establish patient assistance programs to provide financial support or subsidies for eligible patients who cannot afford the treatment.

★ **Government Support:** Government support and funding initiatives can play a crucial role in making the liver cure more accessible to a broader patient population, especially in regions with limited healthcare resources.

★ **International Collaboration:** Collaborations between countries and global health organizations can facilitate access to the liver cure in regions where regulatory approval processes may be more challenging or resource-intensive.

★ **Generic Medications:** If possible, the availability of generic versions of the liver cure can promote competition and drive down prices, making the treatment more affordable for patients.

★ **Advocacy and Awareness:** Patient advocacy groups and healthcare organizations can raise awareness about liver diseases and the importance of access to the liver cure, advocating for policies that support patient access.

★ **Local Manufacturing:** Encouraging local manufacturing of the liver cure in countries with the necessary capabilities can reduce costs and promote access to the treatment.

Patient access and affordability are essential considerations in making the liver cure available to all patients who could benefit from it. By addressing these factors through collaboration, policy support, and patient-focused initiatives, the liver cure's impact can be maximized, positively transforming liver disease management and patient outcomes worldwide.

CHAPTER TEN
FUTURE DEVELOPMENTS AND ONGOING RESEARCH

CHAPTER TEN

FUTURE DEVELOPMENTS AND ONGOING RESEARCH

Future developments and ongoing research in the liver cure hold great promise for advancing liver disease management. Personalized medicine, based on genomics and precision medicine, aims to tailor the liver cure to individual patients for enhanced efficacy and reduced side effects. Combination therapies, combining the liver cure with other treatments, show potential for synergistic effects and improved outcomes. Identifying new therapeutic targets could lead to innovative liver cures for previously challenging conditions. Gene editing and gene therapy offer possibilities for correcting genetic mutations and providing curative treatments. Regenerative medicine explores stem cell therapies and tissue engineering to promote liver tissue repair. Biomarker-based diagnostics aid early detection and monitoring of liver diseases. Artificial intelligence and data analytics expedite analysis of patient data for treatment insights. Long-term safety and efficacy data, along with efforts for global health equity, contribute to improved liver health worldwide. Collaborative efforts among researchers, healthcare providers, and patient advocates will drive advancements, promising a brighter future for liver disease patients.

Expanding Indications

Expanding indications in the liver cure involves systematically investigating its efficacy and safety for a wider range of liver diseases and patient populations. Preclinical studies explore its mechanism of action, while clinical trials assess its effectiveness in diverse liver conditions. Real-world evidence and post-approval surveillance provide valuable data for new indications. Researchers submit supplemental applications to regulatory authorities for approval. This effort addresses unmet medical needs and maximizes the liver cure's impact on liver disease management. Exploration includes rare and pediatric liver diseases, potentially benefiting challenging populations. Combination therapies with other treatments are also investigated to enhance treatment outcomes. International collaboration facilitates approvals in different regions. Supportive health policies encourage research into new liver disease treatments. By continuously expanding indications, the liver cure has the potential to revolutionize liver care, improving outcomes for a broader patient population globally.

Combination Therapies

Combination therapies in the liver cure involve using multiple treatments simultaneously to optimize the management of liver diseases. By targeting different pathways or disease aspects, combination therapies aim to enhance treatment efficacy, reduce resistance, and improve patient outcomes. They offer a personalized approach, considering individual patient profiles and disease stages. The synergy between treatments may lead to better disease control and lower dosages, minimizing side effects.

Clinical trials play a vital role in evaluating the safety and efficacy of combination therapies, providing evidence for their incorporation into routine clinical practice. In liver cancer management, combining surgery, radiation, systemic therapies, and liver-directed treatments shows promise for optimal results.

As research advances, combination therapies hold the potential to revolutionize liver disease treatment, providing more effective and tailored approaches for patients worldwide. However, careful consideration of potential interactions and toxicities remains essential to ensure patient safety and treatment success. Ongoing efforts to refine combination therapy protocols will improve liver disease management, offering hope for better outcomes and improved quality of life for liver disease patients.

CHAPTER ELEVEN

SOCIETAL AND ECONOMIC IMPLICATIONS

Liver diseases have significant societal and economic implications that impact individuals, communities, and healthcare systems. Understanding these implications is essential for addressing the challenges posed by liver diseases and optimizing patient care. **Some key aspects include:**

★ **Healthcare Burden:** Liver diseases place a substantial burden on healthcare systems, including costs related to diagnostics, treatments, hospitalizations, and long-term care. The prevalence of liver diseases and associated healthcare expenses can strain resources and impact the accessibility of healthcare services.

★ **Reduced Productivity:** Liver diseases can lead to decreased workforce participation and reduced productivity due to illness, hospitalization, and treatment-related side effects. This can result in economic losses for individuals, families, and businesses.

★ **Quality of Life:** Liver diseases can significantly impact patients' quality of life, affecting physical well-being, mental health, and social functioning. Addressing these challenges is crucial to improving patients' overall well-being and resilience.

★ **Healthcare Disparities:** Liver diseases can disproportionately affect certain populations, leading to healthcare disparities and unequal access to medical services. Addressing these disparities is vital for promoting health equity and ensuring that all individuals have access to effective liver disease management.

★ **Public Health Initiatives:** Public health initiatives play a vital role in preventing and managing liver diseases, including vaccination campaigns against hepatitis viruses, awareness programs, and lifestyle interventions to address risk factors like alcohol consumption and obesity.

★ **Economic Impact:** Liver diseases' economic consequences include direct healthcare costs, loss of productivity, and indirect costs related to disability and premature mortality. These economic implications highlight the need for effective liver disease management to reduce the burden on individuals and society.

★ **Research and Innovation:** Societal and economic implications underscore the importance of continued research and innovation in liver disease management, seeking novel treatments, preventive strategies, and approaches to reduce the overall impact of liver diseases on society.

Addressing the societal and economic implications of liver diseases requires a comprehensive approach involving healthcare policies, public health initiatives, research investment, and collaborative efforts among stakeholders. By addressing these implications, we can enhance liver disease management, improve patient outcomes, and reduce the overall burden on individuals, communities, and healthcare systems.

Healthcare System Impact

The introduction of the liver cure has a significant impact on healthcare systems worldwide. As a groundbreaking treatment for liver diseases, its implementation brings both challenges and opportunities for healthcare providers, administrators, and policymakers. **Some key aspects of the healthcare system impact in the liver cure include:**

★ **Treatment Accessibility:** Ensuring widespread access to the liver cure requires a coordinated effort to address potential barriers such as cost, insurance coverage, and distribution logistics. Healthcare systems must work to provide equitable access to the treatment for all eligible patients.

★ **Healthcare Costs:** The introduction of the liver cure may initially present financial challenges due to the cost of the treatment. Healthcare systems must carefully evaluate budget allocation and consider cost-effectiveness to optimize its integration while managing overall healthcare expenditures.

★ **Treatment Capacity:** Healthcare facilities must assess their capacity to administer the liver cure, including trained personnel, specialized infrastructure, and diagnostic capabilities, to effectively manage patient demand.

★ **Provider Training:** Healthcare professionals need specialized training to administer the liver cure safely and effectively. Ongoing education and professional development ensure that providers stay updated on the latest advancements and best practices.

★ **Patient Education:** Educating patients about the liver cure, its benefits, potential risks, and treatment expectations is essential for informed decision-making and patient engagement in their care.

★ **Real-World Data Collection:** Monitoring treatment outcomes and safety in real-world settings is crucial for evaluating the liver cure's long-term effectiveness and optimizing patient care.

★ **Healthcare Policies:** Healthcare systems must develop policies and guidelines for the appropriate use of the liver cure, considering patient selection criteria, treatment protocols, and safety monitoring.

★ **Collaborative Efforts:** The successful integration of the liver cure into healthcare systems requires collaboration among healthcare providers, pharmaceutical companies, regulatory authorities, and patient advocacy groups.

While the introduction of the liver cure poses challenges, it also presents opportunities for healthcare systems to improve liver disease management and patient outcomes. By proactively addressing the impact of the liver cure on healthcare systems, stakeholders can work together to optimize its integration, enhance patient care, and transform liver disease management on a global scale.

Cost-Benefit Analysis

Cost-benefit analysis in the liver cure involves evaluating the treatment's economic impact and comparing it to its potential benefits in terms of improved patient outcomes and overall healthcare savings. This analysis is crucial for healthcare systems, policymakers, and stakeholders to make informed decisions regarding the adoption and integration of the liver cure into clinical practice. Key aspects of the cost-benefit analysis include:

★ **Treatment Cost:** The analysis examines the direct costs associated with the liver cure, including the cost of the treatment itself, administration, monitoring, and follow-up care.

★ **Healthcare Savings:** Cost-benefit analysis considers potential healthcare savings resulting from the liver cure's effectiveness in reducing hospitalizations, complications, and the need for other expensive liver disease management interventions.

★ **Improved Patient Outcomes:** Assessing the treatment's impact on patient outcomes, such as reduced morbidity, mortality, and improved quality of life, helps quantify the benefits of the liver cure.

★ **Productivity Gains:** The analysis accounts for potential productivity gains resulting from improved patient health, reduced absenteeism, and increased workforce participation.

★ **Cost-Effectiveness:** Cost-effectiveness analysis examines the liver cure's incremental cost per additional health outcome gained, providing insights into its relative value compared to alternative treatments.

★ **Health Policy Implications:** Cost-benefit analysis informs health policy decisions, considering the financial implications of implementing the liver cure and its potential long-term impact on healthcare systems.

★ **Value-Based Pricing:** The analysis may inform value-based pricing strategies, aligning the cost of the liver cure with its demonstrated clinical benefits and economic value.

★ **Real-World Evidence:** Incorporating real-world evidence into the analysis helps validate the treatment's effectiveness and cost-effectiveness in routine clinical practice.

A comprehensive cost-benefit analysis enables stakeholders to weigh the economic implications of the liver cure against its potential benefits, guiding decisions on treatment adoption, insurance coverage, and healthcare resource allocation. By considering both short-term costs and long-term gains, this analysis supports evidence-based decisions that maximize patient access to effective treatments while ensuring the sustainability of healthcare systems.

Conclusion

In conclusion, the liver cure represents a remarkable advancement in liver disease management in 2023. This groundbreaking treatment offers new hope and opportunities for patients with various liver diseases, revolutionizing their care and improving their quality of life. The comprehensive research and clinical trials leading to its approval have demonstrated the liver cure's efficacy, safety, and potential to transform liver disease outcomes.

As we look ahead, ongoing research and developments continue to enhance our understanding of the liver cure's mechanism of action, its expanding indications, and its integration into healthcare systems worldwide. The combination of personalized medicine, combination therapies, and innovative treatment approaches shows promise in optimizing treatment outcomes for a broad spectrum of liver diseases and diverse patient populations.

The societal and economic implications of the liver cure underscore the need for collaborative efforts among healthcare providers, pharmaceutical companies, regulatory authorities, policymakers, and patient advocacy groups. Together, we can address the challenges posed by liver diseases and work towards achieving health equity and access to this life-changing treatment for all patients in need.

The liver cure's introduction is a testament to the power of scientific innovation and the tireless dedication of the medical community in advancing patient care. As we embrace these exciting developments, we remain committed to continuous research, patient-focused care, and global collaborations, ensuring that the liver cure's impact is felt far beyond 2023, fostering a healthier and brighter future for liver disease patients worldwide.